How to Boost Fertility with Real Food :

A Guide to Preparing Your Body for Pregnancy Through Nutrition and Fertility Awareness. Get Ready to Embrace Parenthood with Confidence!

Barbara J. Winner

Copyright © Barbara J. Winner 2024

Table of contents

Chapter 3
Eating for Fertility: Foods That May Increase Your Chances of Getting Pregnant

Chapter 4
How do menstrual cycles affect fertility?
Understanding the Menstrual Cycle Phases

Chapter 5
What exactly is the concept of tracking fertility?

Chapter 6
How to Enhance Male Fertility and Improve Sperm count

Chapter 7
Exploring Foods that Boost Egg Quality in Women

Chapter 8
Elements Influencing Fertility

Introduction

What Is Fertility?

Fertility refers to the innate ability to have a baby. Not everyone finds conceiving straightforward. Roughly 11% of partnerships encounter infertility, which means they can't get pregnant naturally even after a year of trying without protection. Fertility isn't just a concern for women; it affects individuals of all genders, and there are steps everyone can take to enhance their fertility chances.

Welcoming a child into the world is among the most touching and eagerly anticipated experiences in life. Deciding when to grow your family can be influenced by numerous factors, including meeting the right partner, career timing, financial readiness, emotional preparedness, health status, age, and other family commitments that might postpone the journey to parenthood.

It's common for men and women to spend their early years of fertility avoiding pregnancy. However, once the decision is made to have a child, it seems natural to assume that conception will happen swiftly, ideally within a few months. But if six months go by without success, it's normal to start questioning if there might be a fertility issue at play.

Now, let's talk about the link between a healthy diet and fertility.

If you've been struggling to conceive, it's smart to look at what you're eating. A nutritious diet not only sets the scene for a healthy pregnancy but also lays the groundwork for continued healthy eating into motherhood and beyond. It's a smart move for anyone, no matter how you slice it.

Eating well is crucial for maintaining a healthy body and reproductive system. Research has indicated that a balanced diet and positive lifestyle adjustments can significantly enhance fertility and prime your body for pregnancy. Plus, the lifestyle and dietary choices you make now can impact the quality of sperm and eggs about three months down the line. So, if you're hoping to get pregnant, it's wise to start adopting healthier habits right away.

Chapter 1

What Constitutes Real Food?

Real food is what nature provides. It sprouts from the soil, hangs from branches, roams the plains, or swims in our oceans. It's not concocted in a factory; it's anything that once had a living mother. In essence, real food is alive, and given enough time, it will spoil.

In contrast, "fake" food is heavily processed to last longer on shelves and to appeal to certain consumers (think of who Tony the Tiger is trying to charm). These food pretenders are packed with preservatives, stripped of their natural nutrients, and then, often for marketing reasons, have synthetic nutrients added back in. It's a bit disheartening to realize that so much effort goes into making these items stable, tasty, and visually appealing – to the point where they need to be made to even look like food.

It's said that around 70% of supermarket offerings aren't really food; they're impostors. Our bodies are incredibly adaptable and are built to thrive on real food. Amidst the sea of conflicting dietary advice, one thing stands out: real food is a key to peak performance and warding off illnesses like heart disease, diabetes, obesity, cancer, and depression.

And don't be fooled – real food isn't just about munching on plain fruits and veggies. It's a vast world that includes an array of fruits, vegetables, dairy, eggs, cheese, whole grains, meats of all kinds (yes, even bacon sometimes), seafood, nuts, seeds, natural sweeteners, and much more. The culinary possibilities with real food are endless – think pizzas, burgers, succulent chicken, sandwiches, and a plethora of ethnic dishes. Real food can be simple yet delicious. Once you start feeling the benefits of real food, you might just wonder how you ever got by on those food impostors.

Eating real food seems straightforward, but the abundance of processed, convenient options can make it a challenge. Frozen meals, fast food, and snack packs offer ease but at the cost of flavor and health.

Macronutrients and Fertility

Macronutrients include fats, proteins, and carbohydrates, and getting an adequate balance of these is crucial for preparing the body for conception. Let's dive into how each macronutrient influences fertility and why they're important for increasing the chances of pregnancy.

Protein is vital for building our body's tissues, including everything from collagen to hormones, enzymes, and immune cells. A lack of protein can hinder the body's ability to support the development of another life. It also plays a role in mood regulation, stress reduction, and maintaining balanced blood sugar levels – all of which are important for fertility.

However, not all protein sources are equal, especially when trying to conceive. It's better to avoid proteins that may contain antibiotics, hormones, or heavy metals, often found in animal products. Instead, opt for plant-based proteins like quinoa, organic soy, nuts, beans, and leafy greens, as well as organic, free-range eggs and meats from sustainable sources. Steer clear of processed meats that come with added sugars and unhealthy oils.

Fats are another dietary component that's gotten a bad rap, but they're essential for our health. They protect our organs, keep us warm, help absorb nutrients, and are critical for hormone production. Without fats, our reproductive hormones would be out of balance, potentially leading to infertility. It's important to avoid trans fats and certain vegetable oils that can be inflammatory. Look out for "partially hydrogenated oils" on labels and be wary of products claiming to have zero trans fats – they may still contain harmful amounts.

Incorporate a variety of healthy fats into your diet by choosing foods like extra-virgin olive oil, avocados, avocado oil, coconut oil, nuts, and seeds.

Here's a tip for fellow nut butter enthusiasts: indulge in these creamy delights in moderation, and go for the ones that are purely nuts without added sugars, preservatives, or oils. Or better yet, whip up your own homemade nut butter—it's surprisingly simple!

Carbohydrates serve as the primary energy source for our bodies, fueling everything from our skin to our brain cells. Contrary to some beliefs, carbohydrates themselves aren't inherently fattening. Fiber-rich carbs, in particular, support a healthy digestive system and can assist in the elimination of waste, including excess hormones that might otherwise lead to hormonal imbalances and potential fertility issues.

When choosing carbohydrates, opt for those that can help maintain stable blood sugar levels. Steer clear of highly processed carbs and sugars, such as those found in white flour products, sugary treats, and certain packaged snacks, as they can disrupt insulin balance and may impact fertility.

Good carb choices include whole fruits and vegetables, whole grains and seeds, and oats.

So, what's the ideal balance of macronutrients for a fertility-friendly diet? Aim for a mix of 40% carbohydrates, 25% protein, and 35% fats. This balance is key because both fats and carbs play crucial roles in preparing your body for pregnancy. Adequate carbs prevent your body from conserving energy by shutting down less critical functions, while sufficient fats support hormonal balance and nutrient metabolism, which are essential for reproductive health and growing a new life. Meanwhile, a smaller proportion of protein is necessary for muscle and tissue development.

Chapter 2

Foods to stay away from when trying to conceive.

When you're on the journey to becoming a parent, it's not just about what you should eat to boost your fertility; it's equally important to know which foods might be putting a damper on your efforts. Believe it or not, your diet plays a crucial role in your ability to conceive, and some foods can actually hinder your chances.

The significance of a fertility-friendly diet can't be overstated, especially if you're grappling with challenges like a low sperm count, poor sperm movement, or irregular ovulation, often seen in conditions like PCOS.

What you put on your plate can have a profound impact on both male and female fertility.

So, what's on the no-fly list when you're trying to get pregnant? Let's dive in.

Caffeine can be a bit of a troublemaker, potentially messing with nutrient absorption and increasing the likelihood of miscarriage. It's lurking in your coffee, tea, energy drinks, and chocolate, so it's wise to cut back or cut it out entirely during this time.

Alcohol is another fertility foe. It can throw off your hormonal balance and negatively affect both men's and women's fertility, not to mention increasing the risk of miscarriage and developmental issues in the baby. So, it's best to skip the booze while you're trying to conceive.

Processed foods are not your friends here. They're often packed with unhealthy fats, salt, and sugar, while skimping on the good stuff your body needs to nurture a pregnancy. They can mess with semen quality in guys and ramp up inflammation, which isn't what you want when you're trying to welcome a little one into the world.

High-mercury fish should be avoided, too. Mercury can harm the nervous system, and it's particularly dangerous for developing babies. Stick to safer seafood options like shrimp, pollock, and salmon, which are lower in mercury.

And let's talk fats. Trans fats, saturated fats, and omega-6 fatty acids can stir up inflammation, which is not conducive to conception. You'll find these in processed snacks, some animal products, and certain vegetable oils. Instead, load up on healthy fats like those found in olive oil, avocados, and nuts.

Lastly, those sugary drinks and sodas? They're not doing you any favors. High sugar intake can lead to inflammation and negatively affect egg quality, not to mention its impact on overall organ health, including your reproductive system.

Now, for the good stuff. What should you be munching on while trying to conceive?

Whole, unprocessed foods are the way to go. They're chock-full of essential nutrients like folic acid, iron, and calcium. Make sure you're eating enough calories from a balanced mix of carbs, proteins, and fats to maintain a healthy weight—too much or too little can throw a wrench in your plans.

Protein is key for building the placenta and supporting the baby's growth. Lean meats, beans, and nuts are excellent sources. Folate is another must-have, vital for the baby's neural tube development, so pile your plate with leafy greens and legumes.

Don't forget about iron, which is crucial for increasing blood volume during pregnancy. Lean red meats, poultry, fish, and dark leafy greens are your go-to options here.

By focusing on the right foods and steering clear of the not-so-great ones, you're setting the stage for a healthier pregnancy and boosting your chances of conceiving. It's all about giving your body the best possible foundation to grow a new little life.

To sum it up, adding these superfoods to your meals could potentially tackle infertility issues and give your hormonal and reproductive systems a nice boost:

- Avocados
- Leafy greens that are nice and dark
- All sorts of berries
- A variety of nuts and seeds
- Olive oil that's pure and good
- Whole grains packed with nutrients
- Oily fish, like salmon, that's full of omega-3

When you're on the journey to becoming a parent, what you eat really matters. Certain things on your plate can up the chances of fertility hiccups or complicate things when you're expecting. When you're eager to welcome a little one, it's wise to skip the booze, cut back on the caffeine, say no to processed meats, and steer clear of dairy that hasn't been pasteurized. Stick to a wholesome diet brimming with fresh fruits, veggies, and whole grains to pave the way for a smooth conception and a healthy bump.

Chapter 3

Eating for Fertility: Foods That May Increase Your Chances of Getting Pregnant

The buzz around foods that can potentially enhance fertility is quite popular. However, is there any truth to the idea that certain foods can boost your fertility?

While there's no magic food or diet that guarantees pregnancy, eating a nutritious and balanced diet can play a role in supporting your overall well-being, including your fertility health, for both men and women.

It's crucial to understand that diet alone can't fix all fertility issues. For instance, if a woman has blocked fallopian tubes, no amount of dietary change will clear that blockage.

Keeping this in mind, here's a roundup of 15 wholesome foods that might be helpful for those looking to fine-tune their diet with fertility in mind.

1. Sunflower Seeds

Munch on roasted, unsalted sunflower seed kernels for a vitamin E boost, which might help increase sperm count and movement in some folks. Plus, they're chock-full of folate and selenium, crucial for the fertility of both genders. They're also rich in omega-6 and have some omega-3 fatty acids, which are super important.

Ways to Enjoy Them:
Nibble on sunflower seeds as a snack, sprinkle them on salads, mix them into your trail mix, or swap peanut butter with sunflower seed butter. You can also blend sunflower seed butter into smoothies or stir it into yogurt for an extra kick of flavor and nutrition.

2. Citrus Fruits

Oranges and grapefruits are vitamin C powerhouses. They also have putrescine, a compound that might improve the health of eggs and sperm. However, be cautious with grapefruit if you're on medication, as it can have harmful interactions.

Ways to Enjoy Them:
Snack on orange slices or blend citrus juice into your smoothies. Toss some grapefruit into salads for a zesty twist.

3. Aged Cheeses
Aged cheddar, parmesan, and manchego could be beneficial for sperm health due to their high polyamine content. These proteins, particularly putrescine, might also support egg health, especially in women over 35. But remember, some people might be allergic or intolerant to cheese.

Ways to Enjoy Them:
Add some cheese to your dishes, or enjoy it with nuts or fruit for a snack. Just watch your portions since cheese can be high in saturated fat.

4. Full-Fat Dairy

Full-fat dairy, like whole milk and full-fat yogurt, is great for fertility. A study even suggested women who consume full-fat dairy are less likely to face ovulation issues.

Ways to Enjoy It:

Switch to full-fat dairy options and maybe treat yourself to a serving of full-fat ice cream occasionally, but keep it to once or twice a week.

5. Liver

Cow's liver is incredibly nutrient-dense and offers a wealth of vitamins like A, B12, and other minerals. It's also packed with iron and choline.

Ways to Enjoy It:

Try traditional liver and onions, or sneak liver into meatloaf, shepherd's pie, or meatballs if you're new to it.

6. Cooked Tomatoes
Loaded with the antioxidant lycopene, cooked tomatoes can be beneficial for fertility, especially in men.

Ways to Enjoy Them:
Opt for cooked tomatoes in soups, stews, sauces, or roasted, as they have more lycopene than raw ones.

7. Beans and Lentils
These are fiber and folate-rich, promoting hormonal balance and potentially aiding in egg fertilization due to the polyamine spermidine.

Ways to Enjoy Them:
Use beans or lentils as a meat substitute in meals, or toss them into salads. Choose BPA-free cans if going for canned varieties.

8. Asparagus
This superfood is brimming with vitamin K, folate, and other essential nutrients.

Ways to Enjoy It:
Fresh or frozen asparagus is great roasted, grilled, or added to dishes like frittatas or stir-fries.

9. Oysters

Famous for their fertility-boosting nutrients, oysters are rich in vitamins and minerals like B12, zinc, selenium, and iron.

Ways to Enjoy Them:
Don't be daunted by their preparation; oysters can be eaten raw or baked.

10. Pomegranate

Pomegranates are not only symbolically linked to fertility but are also antioxidant-rich, which may improve sperm quality.

Ways to Enjoy Them:
Enjoy the seeds on their own, or sprinkle them over yogurt, oatmeal, salads, or quinoa bowls.

11

Walnuts are packed with omega-3 and omega-6 fatty acids, which sparked curiosity among scientists about their potential to enhance fertility.

In a fascinating study, 117 men were divided into two groups: one refrained from consuming tree nuts, while the other group enjoyed 75 grams of walnuts each day. Prior to and 12 weeks after the study commenced, the participants provided semen samples.

The walnut-consuming group noticed an uptick in sperm health, including vitality, motility, and morphology, after the 12-week period. They also observed a reduction in chromosomal irregularities in their sperm. The group that abstained from nuts didn't report any changes.

Enjoying Walnuts
Grab a small handful of walnuts for an energizing afternoon nibble. You can also toss them into your chicken salad, morning oatmeal, or even atop a scoop of

ice cream for some nutritious texture. Remember to keep any extra walnuts in the fridge to keep them fresh.

12

Egg Yolks

Egg yolks are the treasure trove of nutrients in eggs, offering nearly all of the iron, calcium, zinc, vitamin B6, folate, and vitamin B12, plus all the vitamin A. Yolks from pasture-raised hens are especially abundant in fertility-enhancing omega-3 fatty acids EPA and DHA, along with vitamins A, D, E, and K2.

Eggs are also a cost-effective lean protein source, which has been linked to improved fertility in both men and women. They're rich in choline too, which may cut down the risk of certain birth defects, although not all research confirms this.

Egg Yolk Consumption

Previously, egg yolks were frowned upon due to cholesterol concerns, but they've since been recognized for their nutrient richness and healthy balance of protein and fats. Eggs are incredibly versatile, so whether you prefer them hard-boiled, scrambled, poached, or fried, go ahead and enjoy the whole egg, yolk and all.

13
Pineapple
There's a popular notion that munching on pineapple core for five days post-ovulation or after an embryo transfer during IVF aids in implantation, but the science doesn't quite support this.

However, pineapples are still worth eating when trying to conceive. They're an excellent vitamin C source, with a single cup serving providing nearly half the daily recommended intake. Low vitamin C has been linked to polycystic ovarian syndrome (PCOS).

Pineapples also boast bromelain, an enzyme with anti-inflammatory and blood-thinning properties, which promotes an immune shift away from inflammation. Since inflammatory foods can hinder fertility and chronic inflammation might inhibit ovulation, this is good news.

Pineapple Enjoyment

Indulge in the natural sweetness of fresh pineapple, as the canning process destroys much of its beneficial bromelain. Eat it by itself, mix it into salsa, or even grill it for a delightful treat.

14

Wild-Caught Salmon

Salmon consistently makes the superfood list, whether for general health or fertility, thanks to its abundance of essential fatty acids and omega-3s, which are known to support fertility. It's also a fish with low mercury levels.

Salmon is also rich in selenium and vitamin D, both crucial for healthy sperm and overall fertility. Just a 3-ounce serving of smoked salmon provides nearly all the daily recommended vitamin D intake.

Salmon Serving Suggestions

When trying to conceive or during pregnancy, it's essential to be mindful of mercury levels in fish. Opt for wild-caught salmon over farm-raised to avoid mercury, antibiotics, and artificial food dyes.

15

Cinnamon

For women with polycystic ovarian syndrome (PCOS), a leading cause of infertility, taking cinnamon supplements may help kickstart irregular menstrual cycles. But before you reach for supplements, consider integrating cinnamon into your diet.

In a small yet notable study, women with PCOS who took a daily cinnamon supplement reported almost double the number of menstrual cycles compared to those on a placebo. More regular ovulatory cycles increase the chances of conception.

Cinnamon Consumption

Sprinkle some cinnamon on your oatmeal, yogurt, or into your tea or coffee for a flavorful boost. While cinnamon supplements are an option, it's wise to consult with your healthcare provider before beginning any new supplement regimen.

Chapter 4

How do menstrual cycles affect fertility?

When you're planning for a baby, a missed period is often the first hint of pregnancy many women look for. This fact alone highlights the deep connection between menstrual cycles and fertility, yet there's much more to this relationship than just an indicator of pregnancy success or lack thereof.

A missed period might suggest pregnancy, but it's not a certainty. Sometimes, a missed period can point to amenorrhea, which may be due to factors like low body weight, stress, intense exercise, or conditions such as polycystic ovary syndrome (PCOS), potentially leading to infertility rather than pregnancy.

In this section, we'll dive into how your period impacts your chances of conceiving and tackle some common queries to deepen your understanding of your menstrual cycle.

What Does a Missed Period Indicate?

A missed period could mean various things, from pregnancy to fertility issues. An expert gynecologist can pinpoint the cause through tests or check-ups.

How can you tell if you've missed a period? It's straightforward: count the days from the start of your last period to the beginning of the next one. A typical cycle spans 21 to 35 days, though it can vary. If you don't get your period after 35 days, it might be delayed or missed.

Reasons for a missed period include:

Pregnancy – as mentioned, this could be why your period hasn't shown up.

Stress – a common culprit, especially when anxious about conceiving.

Body weight extremes – being underweight can halt ovulation, while obesity can disrupt hormones and menstruation.

PCOS – a prevalent condition marked by hormonal imbalances and irregular periods.

Chronic illnesses – conditions like coeliac disease and diabetes can affect periods.

Birth control changes – starting or stopping hormonal birth control can lead to irregular periods.

Thyroid issues – an imbalanced thyroid can impact weight and hormones, affecting periods.

Less common causes include early menopause, pituitary tumors, and ectopic pregnancy.

Period Intensity and Fertility: Is There a Link?

Light periods don't necessarily mean reduced fertility, but they can make conceiving harder if they indicate a thin uterine lining, which is less conducive to egg implantation.

Heavy periods don't equate to higher fertility either. Instead, they might signal conditions like endometriosis, which can interfere with fertility.

Spotting between periods could be due to hormonal imbalances or physical conditions and doesn't always suggest a serious problem. Sometimes, it's just due to minor causes like dryness or vigorous intercourse. Spotting can also be an early pregnancy sign.

Regular periods are a positive sign for fertility, but normal cycles don't guarantee it. Other factors like STIs or your partner's fertility could play a role.

Is Pregnancy Possible Right After Your Period?

Yes, though it's less likely, you can conceive right after your period, especially with a short cycle and early ovulation. Since sperm can survive in the body for up to seven days, it's wise to have sex throughout your cycle when trying to conceive and use protection consistently if you're not.

Understanding the Menstrual Cycle Phases

The menstrual cycle's goal is to prepare for pregnancy, with each cycle varying in length and intensity.

The cycle has four phases:

1. Menstrual phase: When you get your period, the uterus sheds its lining as the unfertilized egg from the previous cycle didn't lead to pregnancy, causing hormone levels to drop.

2. Follicular phase: Overlapping with the menstrual phase, it lasts until ovulation, with FSH from the pituitary gland stimulating the ovaries to produce follicles, leading to one mature egg and a thickened uterine lining.

3. Ovulation phase: Triggered by rising estrogen and LH, a mature egg is released and ready for fertilization,

indicated by symptoms like a slight temperature rise and thicker discharge.

4. Luteal phase: Post-ovulation, the focus is on maintaining the uterine lining in case of pregnancy; if not, the cycle restarts.

Remember, the length of each phase can vary throughout your life.

Did you realize that because sperm can survive inside the female body for up to five days, it's possible for pregnancy to occur from intercourse that happens as many as five days prior to ovulation?

Let's talk about the luteal phase. Once the egg is released by the follicle, it transforms into the corpus luteum, a hormone-secreting body that primarily pumps out progesterone and a bit of estrogen. These hormones are crucial because they keep the lining of your uterus thick, providing a cozy spot for a fertilized egg to settle down.

If pregnancy does happen, your body will start producing human chorionic gonadotropin (hCG), which is the hormone those pregnancy tests look for. It's like a support system for the corpus luteum, ensuring the uterine lining stays plush.

But if pregnancy isn't in the cards, the corpus luteum will shrink and eventually get reabsorbed, leading to a drop in hormone levels, and voilà, your period begins, and the uterine lining is shed.

During the luteal phase, if you aren't expecting, you might notice some premenstrual syndrome (PMS) symptoms like bloating, breast changes, mood swings, headaches, weight gain, shifts in libido, food cravings, and sleep issues. This phase typically lasts between 11 to 17 days, with 14 days being the average.

Now, let's chat about spotting menstrual cycle issues. Everyone's cycle has its own rhythm; some are like clockwork, while others are more unpredictable. The heaviness and duration of bleeding can also vary.

Life stages can stir things up too. For instance, as menopause approaches, your cycle might get a bit erratic.

One handy tip for keeping tabs on your cycle is to jot down when your periods start and end, along with any changes in flow or unexpected spotting.

Here are some things that can shake up your menstrual cycle:

- Birth control can make your periods lighter and shorter, or sometimes make them vanish altogether.
- Pregnancy brings a halt to your periods, and a missed period is often the first clue that you might be pregnant.
- Polycystic ovary syndrome (PCOS) messes with egg development and can lead to irregular or missed periods.
- Uterine fibroids can extend and amplify your periods.

- Eating disorders can throw your cycle out of whack and even cause your periods to stop.

Here are some red flags that there might be an issue with your menstrual cycle:

- Skipping periods or a complete stop of periods.
- Unpredictable periods.
- Bleeding that goes on for more than a week.
- Periods that are too close together or too far apart.
- Bleeding between periods that's more than just light spotting.

If you're experiencing these or any other menstrual concerns, it's a good idea to have a chat with a healthcare provider.

Remember, menstrual cycles are as unique as you are. Knowing your own cycle well, including the timing and duration of your periods, is key. Stay vigilant for any changes and don't hesitate to discuss them with a healthcare pro.

Chapter 5

What exactly is the concept of tracking fertility?

Can anyone track their fertility?

What are the perks of keeping tabs on fertility?

What are the drawbacks of monitoring fertility?

What varieties of fertility tracking exist?

Understanding your fertility involves recognizing the days during your cycle when you're most likely to get pregnant. You can use this knowledge for birth control or to increase your chances of conception.

This practice goes by various names, such as natural family planning, and it can be done through multiple methods like the symptothermal approach, the ovulation technique, periodic abstinence, the mucus strategy, the Billings method, and the rhythm method.

For roughly half of your monthly cycle, pregnancy isn't in the cards. By observing signs of ovulation, such as changes in body temperature or vaginal mucus, you can gauge your fertile windows. Avoiding intercourse on these days lessens the likelihood of pregnancy.

Fertility tracking demands meticulous adherence to guidelines—and your partner's full cooperation. Since conception is possible a few days before and after ovulation, it's crucial to abstain from sex during this window.

The six-day span that includes the five days leading up to ovulation and the day it occurs is when you're most fertile. Sperm can survive inside you for up to five days, so intercourse during this time can result in pregnancy.

Post-ovulation, an egg only survives for 12 to 24 hours. Once this period lapses, the opportunity for pregnancy is over until the next cycle.

Can anyone track their fertility?
Fertility tracking might not be the best fit if:

You've recently stopped hormonal birth control, like the pill.
Your menstrual cycles are irregular.
You're nearing menopause.
Your partner isn't fully on board.

What are the perks of keeping tabs on fertility?
The benefits of fertility tracking include its natural, side-effect-free approach to birth control. It's an ideal

option for those who, for religious, cultural, or health reasons, prefer not to use other contraceptives.

When followed correctly and with strong commitment to preventing pregnancy, it can be quite effective. It's cost-free and promotes intimate knowledge of your body.

What are the drawbacks of monitoring fertility?
One of the cons of using fertility tracking as a contraceptive is the higher chance of unintended pregnancy compared to other methods. Success hinges on your diligence in following the method. Statistically, about 1 in 4 women practicing this method may become pregnant.

It requires time, patience, and strict adherence to guidelines. Even then, predicting ovulation can be tricky for some.

Fertility tracking methods won't shield you from sexually transmitted infections (STIs). For STI protection, you'll need to use additional methods like condoms.

Also, factors like illness, stress, certain medications, or sexual activity can influence the accuracy of fertility tracking.

What varieties of fertility tracking exist?
Different strategies exist for using fertility tracking to prevent pregnancy:

Cervical Mucus or Billings Method
Your vaginal mucus changes throughout the month. After your period, you may notice dryness, then around ovulation, the mucus becomes clear and stretchy. Once ovulation passes, it gets thicker. These changes help pinpoint ovulation. Avoid intercourse until three dry days have occurred.

This method may not be suitable if you experience abnormal vaginal bleeding, have cervical or vaginal inflammation, or are on medications like antibiotics that alter your mucus.

Temperature Method

A slight increase in your resting temperature indicates ovulation. You'll need to measure your temperature daily before getting out of bed. Once your temperature has risen for three consecutive days, you're clear to have intercourse for the next few days.

However, this isn't the most reliable method since numerous factors can affect your temperature. It also limits intercourse to about 12 days in a 28-day cycle.

Symptothermal Method

Combine morning temperature readings with evening cervical mucus checks to determine safe days for intercourse.

Additional ovulation signs to watch for include mild cramps, spotting, and breast tenderness. Using multiple indicators together enhances the accuracy of fertility tracking.

Calendar or Rhythm Method
This approach is less reliable, especially for those with irregular cycles. You can learn more about calendar-based methods through resources like Family Planning NSW.

Chapter 6

How to Enhance Male Fertility and Improve Sperm count

Enhancing male fertility and raising sperm count can be achieved through an active lifestyle, reducing stress, and adopting dietary and lifestyle modifications.

If you and your partner are facing fertility challenges, remember that this is a common issue. Approximately one out of six couples encounter infertility, and in about a third of these cases, the problem lies with the male partner.

While not all infertility issues can be addressed, there are measures you can take to improve your odds of conceiving. A nutritious diet, certain supplements, and lifestyle adjustments can sometimes enhance fertility.

This section highlights key lifestyle elements, foods, nutrients, and supplements linked to better fertility in men.

What does male infertility mean?
The ability to conceive naturally is what we refer to as fertility.

Male infertility is the diminished likelihood of a man being able to impregnate his female partner, often related to the quality of his sperm cells.

Infertility can be associated with sexual function or semen quality. Here are a few examples:

- Libido: Also known as sex drive, libido is the desire to engage in sexual activity. Substances that are believed to boost libido are known as aphrodisiacs.
- Erectile dysfunction: Also called impotence, it's the inability of a man to achieve or maintain an erection.

- Sperm count: A key aspect of semen quality is the number or concentration of sperm in a given amount of semen.
- Sperm motility: The ability of sperm to swim effectively, which is crucial for fertility.
- Testosterone levels: Low levels of testosterone, the male sex hormone, can be linked to infertility in some men.

Infertility can stem from various factors, including genetics, overall health, physical condition, diseases, and exposure to dietary contaminants.

Moreover, a healthy lifestyle and diet are crucial. Certain foods and nutrients offer more fertility benefits than others.

Here are 10 scientifically supported methods to enhance sperm count and boost fertility in men.

1. Consider D-aspartic acid supplements

D-aspartic acid (D-AA) is an amino acid sold as a dietary supplement, not to be confused with the more common L-aspartic acid.

D-AA is found primarily in certain glands, like the testicles, and in semen and sperm cells.

Studies suggest that D-AA plays a role in male fertility, as levels are typically lower in infertile men. D-AA supplements have been shown to increase testosterone levels, crucial for fertility.

For instance, one study indicated that taking 2.7 grams of D-AA for three months raised testosterone by 30–60% and sperm count and motility by 60–100%, leading to more pregnancies in their partners.

Another study found that 3 grams of D-AA daily for two weeks boosted testosterone by 42%. However, results are mixed, and more research is needed to determine the long-term effects and benefits of D-AA supplements in humans.

2. Regular exercise

Regular physical activity not only benefits your overall health but can also raise testosterone levels and improve fertility.

Research has shown that active men have higher testosterone levels and better semen quality than inactive men. However, excessive exercise may have the opposite effect, potentially lowering testosterone levels. Adequate zinc intake can mitigate this risk.

If you're not very active but want to improve your fertility, prioritizing physical activity is essential.

3. Sufficient vitamin C intake

Vitamin C is well-known for its immune-boosting effects.

Some research suggests that antioxidant supplements, like vitamin C, could enhance fertility.

Oxidative stress occurs when there's an imbalance between reactive oxygen species (ROS) and the body's ability to detoxify them or repair the resulting damage.

Excessive ROS can lead to tissue damage, inflammation, and increased risk of chronic disease. It's also implicated in male infertility.

Antioxidants like vitamin C may help mitigate these effects. Studies have shown that vitamin C supplements can improve semen quality, with one study showing a 92% increase in sperm motility and more than a 100% increase in sperm count, as well as a significant reduction in deformed sperm cells.

These findings suggest vitamin C could improve fertility in men with oxidative stress, but more research is necessary for conclusive claims.

4. Reduce stress

Stress can hinder your mood for intimacy, but it might also impact fertility more directly. Stress is believed to affect fertility through the hormone cortisol.

Long-term stress can increase cortisol, which negatively impacts testosterone. When cortisol rises, testosterone often decreases.

Stress can be managed through various techniques like nature walks, meditation, exercise, or socializing.

5. Adequate vitamin D

Vitamin D is vital for both male and female fertility and may help increase testosterone levels.

Observational studies have shown that vitamin D deficiency is linked to low testosterone levels. A study found that taking 3,000 IU of vitamin D3 daily for a year increased testosterone levels by about 25%.

Higher vitamin D levels are associated with better sperm motility, although research results vary.

6. Try tribulus terrestris
Tribulus terrestris, also known as puncture vine, is an herb used to boost male fertility.

One study found that taking 6 grams of tribulus root daily for two months improved erectile function and sex drive.

Although Tribulus terrestris doesn't increase testosterone levels, it may enhance the libido-promoting effects of testosterone. More research is required to confirm its benefits and potential long-term effects.

7. Fenugreek supplements
Fenugreek is a common culinary and medicinal herb.

Research has shown that taking 500 mg of fenugreek extract daily can increase testosterone levels, strength, and fat loss. Another study demonstrated improved libido, sexual performance, and testosterone levels with a 600 mg daily dose of a fenugreek-based supplement.

However, these studies focused on extracts, and whole fenugreek used in cooking or tea might not be as effective.

8. Sufficient zinc intake
Zinc is a vital mineral found in high amounts in animal products like meat, fish, eggs, and shellfish.

Incorporating these methods into your daily routine can potentially enhance your fertility and increase your chances of conception.

Maintaining adequate zinc levels is crucial for men's reproductive health. Research has found that insufficient zinc can lead to lower testosterone levels, subpar sperm quality, and a heightened risk of infertility in men.

Moreover, zinc supplementation has been shown to elevate testosterone levels and increase sperm count for those with zinc deficiencies.

It's also interesting to note that zinc can help mitigate the testosterone reduction often seen in athletes following intense workout regimens.

However, we should keep in mind that these observations need to be verified through rigorous clinical trials.

Now, let's talk about ashwagandha, also known as Withania somnifera. This ancient herb from India is reputed for its positive effects on male fertility, including a potential boost in testosterone.

One particular study observed men with low sperm counts and found that daily intake of 675 mg of ashwagandha root extract over three months led to a remarkable improvement in fertility, with sperm counts skyrocketing by 167%, semen volume by 53%, and sperm motility by 57%. Those on a placebo saw only minor changes.

These fertility enhancements might be partly due to the rise in testosterone. For example, young men undergoing strength training and consuming 600 mg of ashwagandha root extract daily experienced significant gains in testosterone levels, muscle mass, and strength, unlike those who took a placebo.

Observational studies back up these claims, suggesting that ashwagandha supplements can increase sperm counts, motility, antioxidant levels, and testosterone.

Moving on to maca root, this Peruvian plant is famed for its ability to boost libido, fertility, and overall sexual function.

Men consuming between 1.5 to 3 grams of dried maca root over a few months reported heightened sexual desire. Additionally, for those with mild erectile issues, 2.4 grams of dried maca root over 12 weeks showed a slight improvement in erectile function and sexual well-being.

Healthy men taking 1.75 grams of maca root powder daily for three months also saw an uptick in sperm count and motility.

While these findings are promising, reviews suggest that the evidence is not conclusive, and further studies are necessary to solidify these claims. Also, it's worth noting that maca root doesn't seem to impact hormone levels, as no changes in testosterone or other reproductive hormones were observed in healthy men after taking maca root for three months.

Chapter 7

Exploring Foods that Boost Egg Quality in Women

Navigating the complex world of fertility, a woman's egg quality is essential for conception success. We'll dive into how nutrition influences reproductive health and spotlight foods that can potentially improve egg quality—an often overlooked yet vital piece of the conception puzzle. From understanding how egg health works to actionable diet and lifestyle tips, we're about to empower women with the tools to nurture their eggs with nature's gifts.

Demystifying Female Egg Quality

What's Egg Quality All About?
Egg quality is crucial for fertility. It's about the egg's genetic integrity and its ability to be fertilized.

Influenced by age, genetics, and lifestyle, egg quality is something we can support with lifestyle changes, especially through our diets.

Nutrition's Role in Egg Quality

Our diet does more than satisfy hunger—it's fundamental for reproductive health. It shapes our hormone balance, supports cellular processes, and helps fight oxidative stress. Every nutrient is a key player in the reproductive system's symphony.

Think of your body as a delicate instrument, with nutrients as the strings that create a harmonious hormonal tune. The vitamins, minerals, and antioxidants in our food are the building blocks, setting the stage for fertility to thrive. These nutritional architects are crafting a fertile environment, influencing our eggs' DNA.

We wield the power to shape our reproductive wellness with our dietary choices. The vegetables, grains, and omega-3-rich fish we consume all contribute to a masterpiece that could improve our eggs' quality. Each meal is a brushstroke on our reproductive journey, a reminder that our plate's choices can brighten our future.

Key Nutrients for Better Egg Quality
Antioxidants: Egg Protectors
Antioxidants combat oxidative stress, which can harm egg quality. Berries, leafy greens, and nuts like almonds and walnuts are antioxidant powerhouses that protect our eggs from damage.

Omega-3s: Hormonal Harmony
Known for their anti-inflammatory effects and hormone regulation, omega-3s are found in fatty fish and plant sources like flaxseeds. They help maintain a balanced hormonal environment for healthy egg development.

Folate: DNA's Best Friend
Folate is crucial for DNA repair and synthesis. Dark greens, avocados, and lentils, rich in folate, help preserve your egg's genetic material.

Vitamin D: Reproductive Health Booster

Vitamin D influences hormone levels and menstrual cycles. Sunlight and vitamin D-rich foods like fatty fish and fortified dairy are key for healthy eggs.

Iron: Oxygenating the Reproductive System
Iron ensures tissues, including reproductive organs, are well-oxygenated. Red meat, beans, and spinach are great iron sources, promoting optimal blood flow and egg health.

B Vitamins: Energy for Eggs
B vitamins are vital for energy metabolism. A diet with whole grains, lean meats, and greens supplies B vitamins, supporting energy and healthy egg development.

Plant-Based Foods for Egg Vitality
Phytoestrogens: Hormonal Balance
Phytoestrogens in foods like soy, flaxseeds, and legumes may help maintain hormonal balance, supporting reproductive health.

Colorful Produce: Antioxidant Riches
The antioxidants in colorful fruits and veggies fight oxidative stress, potentially boosting egg quality and reducing inflammation.

Whole Grains: Fiber's Role
Whole grains offer fiber, which helps stabilize blood sugar and supports hormonal balance—important for egg health.

Lifestyle Tips for Egg Quality
Exercise: Beyond Weight
Regular, balanced exercise helps regulate hormones and improve blood circulation, fostering the right conditions for egg development.

Stress Management: Clearing the Clouds
Chronic stress can upset hormonal balance and egg quality. Mindfulness and self-care can help manage stress, creating a more fertile environment.

Superfoods for Egg Excellence

Royal Jelly: Nutrient-Rich
Royal jelly is packed with fertility-supporting nutrients. Consult a healthcare provider before adding it to your diet.

Maca Root: Hormonal Equilibrium
Maca root is thought to promote hormonal balance and support menstrual regularity. Approach its use mindfully and seek medical advice.

Spirulina: The Green Dynamo
Spirulina is a superfood with potential health benefits, including for reproduction. Its antioxidant power fights oxidative stress, but be sure to get professional advice before diving in.

Crafting a Fertility-Friendly Diet
A Day of Fertility-Boosting Meals
Imagine starting with a berry and spinach smoothie with flaxseed and Greek yogurt. Lunch could be a vibrant salad with protein and diverse veggies. Dinner might star

grilled salmon with quinoa and steamed broccoli. Snack on almonds or fruit during the day.

Simple Steps for Better Egg Quality

Embarking on a journey to boost egg quality doesn't have to be daunting. Making small tweaks to what you eat and how you live can make a big difference over time. Teaming up with a health expert or a dietitian can offer you advice that's just right for you.

Personalized Eating for Fertility

When it comes to fertility, there's this idea of tailoring what you eat to suit your body's genetic makeup and health condition. By getting to know your genetic makeup and what your body needs, you can get diet advice that's spot-on for improving egg quality. A diet that's customized for you can fix any nutrient shortages, help your body get the most out of the food you eat, and reduce the impact of any genetic factors that might be affecting your fertility. Knowing which nutrients are key for making healthy eggs can help you make the best choices for your reproductive health.

This way of personalizing your diet helps you match what you eat with your body's genetic and health profile, which might boost your chances of having better egg quality.

Best Ways to Cook for Keeping Nutrients
When you're trying to keep all the good stuff in your food, especially for fertility, it's all about cooking gently. Techniques like steaming, light sautéing, and slow cooking help keep the nutrients that are good for fertility. Steaming veggies keeps their vitamins, and cooking with just a little oil keeps the nutrients in. Cooking slowly at lower temperatures keeps the important nutrients strong for reproductive health.

These cooking methods make sure that the food you eat for fertility keeps all its nutritional benefits, helping you make smart, healthy choices in the kitchen.

Eating a Variety for Fertility

Having a wide-ranging diet is super important for fertility and staying healthy in general. Try lots of different foods and flavors to make sure you're getting all sorts of nutrients. Eating a mix of things, like colorful veggies, lean proteins, and whole grains, lays a solid foundation for what your body needs.

This mix isn't just good for fertility; it also strengthens your overall health. Think of trying new foods as a way to feed your body well, which can help your chances of having good fertility and health.

Why Regular Health Checks Matter

Keeping up with regular health checks is crucial for keeping an eye on your fertility. These check-ups can give you really useful info, helping you make changes early on that can have a big effect on your fertility. Doctors can spot little changes, sort out any issues, and give you advice that's meant just for you. By keeping on top of these visits, you're arming yourself with knowledge about your fertility.

Staying on top of your health like this means you can tweak your lifestyle, what you eat, or get treatments if needed, setting you on a path to better egg quality and a better chance of getting pregnant.

Chapter 8

Elements Influencing Fertility

The age of a woman is a crucial element influencing fertility. From birth, the amount of eggs a woman has dwindles daily. Younger women lose eggs slowly, but the decline accelerates after their mid-30s, leading to fewer eggs and a higher chance of miscarriage if pregnancy occurs.

Men's fertility may also dip with age, but not as significantly.

Having had a previous pregnancy boosts a couple's chances of conceiving again, regardless of the previous pregnancy's outcome.

The longer a couple has been trying to conceive without success, the lower their chances become. Those trying for under three years have a better shot than those trying for longer.

The timing and frequency of sexual activity are key. A typical menstrual cycle lasts 28 days, with ovulation on day 14. The best chance to conceive is having sex two days before ovulation. Regular sexual activity, about 2-3 times a week, ensures plenty of fresh sperm is available for fertilization.

Lifestyle choices also play a role.

Excess weight can lead to irregular menstrual cycles and reduced ovulation, making it harder to conceive. Losing even a small percentage of body weight can improve menstrual regularity and fertility. Men with excess weight might have less optimal sperm.

Conversely, being underweight can also hinder fertility by disrupting regular ovulation. Gaining weight can help improve fertility.

Smoking can triple the time it takes to get pregnant and harm the reproductive system in both women and men. It decreases a woman's ovarian reserve and can damage sperm quality in men.

Caffeine doesn't have a clear link to infertility.

Alcohol consumption is a bit of a mixed bag, with some studies showing that over five units a week may reduce fertility, while others suggest moderate drinking could be linked to higher pregnancy rates. However, it's advised to avoid alcohol when trying to conceive due to potential risks.

Over-the-counter and recreational drugs can interfere with various reproductive functions, from ovulation to sperm production.

Lastly, certain medical conditions like thyroid disease, vitamin D deficiency, polycystic ovary syndrome, and endometriosis can impact fertility. Some might be known before trying to conceive, while others might be diagnosed during the process.